DIE NO MORE

Ralph Milione, B.S.PH

ISBN:1481872125
ISBN-13:9781481872126

DEDICATION

I dedicate this book to my patient, understanding wife Marie and to my children Victor, Patricia and Clare and to my daughter in law Janet and my grandchildren Lauren and Ryan for encouraging me to finish this book.

CONTENTS

THE PHARMACIST`S PRAYER

O Divine and Holy Spirit of Love, look down upon Thy humble servant to whom are confided the lives of human beings. Deign to be my light guide, my strength and all the Love of my heart. Be my courage when I must stand by the laws of God and morality. Never let me be guilty of the moral decrepitation of my human being. Let me rather be an inspiration to my fellow men in their hour of trial and need.

Take from me selfishness, softness, cowardice and fear. Give me the spirit of endurance and firmness love of labor, silence and charity. Make me always responsive to Thy Holy Inspiration that if it be Thy Holy Will, I might bring help strength to the suffering members of Your mystical Body.

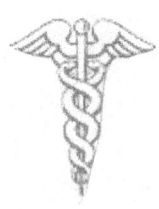

FORWARD

The reason I wrote this book was because over the past 35 years as a practicing pharmacist I came across a question asked by many of my customers regarding the most fearful word CANCER and how to prolong life. What are the most important factors necessary for man to stay healthy? Is it possible for man to live forever? Can we overcome all sickness and disease known to man? Can modern doctors and scientist discover the secret to longevity for all mankind? Can CANCER be eliminated completely in our lifetime?

In writing this book I have compiled the data I have accumulated over the years on CANCER and other important factors which will enlighten the reader and bring a better understanding of CANCER.

I believe within our time we will see all diseases being cured and man will live forever. We have made great strides in the research of cures for many once incurable diseases and today many have been eradicated with great success with the discovery of genes, DNA, and chromosomes where telomeres can be extended.

We are on the threshold of discovery, just beginning a new approach to man's immortality. Will we live forever in the foreseeable future? The information presented herein will give you a much better understanding of how man can prove life can be extended to infinity providing enough effort and research is administered by the medical profession and scientists who believe man can achieve immortality.

Telomeres which are the junk DNA strains at the end of each chromosome keep the chromosomes together and protect the chromosomes from breaking up. As one grows older, the strands break off and the telomeres shorten. The shorter the telomeres the older one becomes. This is where the telomerase enzyme comes in to prevent telomeres from shortening. Since the discovery of telomerase enzyme, scientist have been successful in preventing telomeres from shortening thereby preventing ageing and extending one's life well beyond 100 and even into infinity.

In the following pages I have listed a few procedures which explain methods to prevent cancer and have been shown to be successful with cancer patients.

1 FDA

The Federal Drug Administration was set up by the government to protect the public's health by assuring the safety, efficacy and security of human and veterinary drugs, biological products medical devices, our nation's food supply, cosmetics and products that emit radiation. Also responsible for advancing the public health by helping speed innovations that make medicines more effectively safer and more affordable by helping the public get the accurate scientific basic information they need to use medicines and foods in maintaining and improving health. In addition the FDA also has responsibility for regulating the manufacturing, marketing and distribution of tobacco products to protect the public health and to reduce tobacco use by minors. This statement can be found on the FDA website.

According to "Life Extension" book published in 2009 by Praktikos Books, "Americans are prescribed drugs whose approval may be based on fraudulent or insufficient research data. Experimental therapies that could save lives are routinely denied."

There are some other important facts which might enlighten you the reader regarding the FDA. The FDA speak the gospel truth but appear to do just the opposite as proven by a statement made by the FDA commissioner Dr. Eschenbach who issued a sixty page report entitled, "FDA Science and Mission". Following are his exact quotes:

> "The FDA cannot fulfill its mission because its scientific base has eroded and its scientific organizational structure is weak. The FDA cannot fulfill its mission because its scientific work force does not have sufficient capacity and capability. The FDA cannot fulfill its mission because its information technology (IT) infrastructure is inadequate. The FDA does not have the capacity to ensure the safety of food for the nation."

Where does this leave us? Here we have a confession by the Commissioner who states the FDA is not capable of filling its duties as a viable agency and now we are left with the uncertainties of whether the drugs which are on the market are safe for human consumption. If a doctor recommends a drug for our sickness and it is approved by the FDA are we sure the drug is not toxic? Can we be sure of anything the FDA states in the future? Should the FDA be revamped, dismantled and started anew? From the FDA's indictment of itself are we to believe the food, air and water we consume and breath is safe?

This is a Catch 22, if we choose to eat fruit, vegetables, meat, fish chicken and other products, can we be certain they will not make us sickly or are free of toxic chemicals?

The reason I included the topic on the FDA is that the reader should be aware that our food supplies, air and water are not being supervised nor inspected annually by the FDA. It will be upon us to petition our Representatives to make our demands heard.

I personally telephoned the FDA and inquired as to how often American farms are inspected by the FDA. I was told once every ten years! How often are drug companies and restaurants inspected? They told me they don't have the resources or financial means to survey these establishments. I asked when a product is submitted to the FDA for approval does the FDA have their own chemists, doctors, research technicians to examine the product? They answered "they are not set up to reexamine products but make their decision on the pharmaceutical companies research data presented".

This means if the pharmaceutical chemist's research reports show somewhat of a very small benefit then the drug is approved. Yet if there is some form of toxicity shown it is not reported. The FDA will only take the product off the market when it is deemed unsafe for public use. Another fact is when the product kills five thousand people the FDA warns the big drug companies to take the item off the market and gives them a penalty of 4.5 billion dollars with the understanding a black box label must be applied to their products, warning the consumer of its toxicity.

The drug company is left manufacturing other highly questionable drugs. The drug company's statement to the FDA is they are unable to remove their condemned drug because the drug is sold worldwide and it would take five to ten years before it can be completely removed. Here we will see the drug will continue to be sold and will also continue to kill people.

This is a crime against humanity and a crime against Americans who have given their trust to the FDA. The most important issue today is the FDA must be reorganized and supervised by the government to ensure the FDA lives up to its bylaws.

2 CANCER

Cancer is a controversial subject today with leading oncologists. Some believe there is a cure for Cancer, others believe there is not. If you believe modern day drugs are the answers than you are wrong, for drugs will not cure Cancer. Drugs may hold back the spread of Cancer but only for a limited time. Before making a final decision as to whether to undergo Cancer treatment, get a second opinion and even a third opinion for you have only one body make sure you take good care it.

If someone is diagnosed as being in the fourth stages of Cancer, they should look into alternative therapies to be used with orthodox treatments for Cancer.

Here is listed a therapy and a compound which is being used today in the treatment of Lung, Prostate, and Melanomas.

GLIOBLASTOMA

A study, financed by Novo Cure which is a private founded company in Israel, was made in the U.S. and Europe to use electricity to kill cancer cells. Electrical currents are attached to the brain which send currents into the cancer cells and shake them apart. The good cells are not affected. Today this treatment is being used for Lung Cancer patients in some U.S. hospitals and there have had good results. These methods are also being used as experimental these methods of treatment for kidney and bladder Cancers.

If someone you know is suffering from Glioblastoma (brain cancer) there is a good video you can watch on Novacure-www.Bill Doyle.com. This concerns treating brain cancer with electrical fields.

DAMMARANE SAPOGENINES

Dammarane Sapogenines are a group of compounds found in plants and have been used in China for many years. They do show much Cancer killing activity per se, yet it is used to strengthen the immune system whereby helping the T, and B-Cells kill off Cancer cells. Ginseng is a series of natural nontoxic herbal products which is formulated to contain mainly dammarane sapogenines. In conjunction with Cancer therapies it has been shown to reduce nausea and stomach pains when undergoing treatments for Cancer.

It is being used and has been used for years in Asia to increase mental performance and to help when dealing with stressful situations. It will also strengthen the body's organs against environmental pollutants and has been found to kill a very wide range of cancer cells of different origins of different backgrounds. It can be used to treat Prostate and pancreatic Cancers.

It is being used and has been used for years in Asia to increase mental performance and to help when dealing with stressful situations. It will also strengthen the body's organs against environmental pollutants and has been found to kill a very wide range of cancer cells of different origins of different backgrounds. It can be used to treat Prostate and pancreatic Cancers.

Before taking this compound discuss it with your oncologist to know if it is right for you. Even though it might not have any dangerous side effects protect yourself no matter what drugs or herbs you are taking. Remember all drugs are dangerous and have side effects.   This product can be purchased from the Careseng Wellness TCM Centre in Richmond B.C.Canada.

STAGES OF CANCER

There are four stages of cancer- Stages 1, 2, 3 4.

Stage 1-The cancer has progressed to the connective tissues.

Stage 2-The cancer has turned into a tumor and has grown into the muscle's layers.

Stage 3-The cancer has continued to spread into the muscle layers and into the fatty tissues of the body.

Stage 4-The cancer has spread into the lymph nodes and throughout the entire body.

When a person is diagnosed they are in stage 1. This is the time to start treating the body with complementary therapies starting with the therapies I have outlined earlier in treating the entire body. Follow a change of diet, changing one's lifestyle, proper nutrition, vitamin therapy, exercising, meditation, stress free life and being optimistic in life; regulating caloric intake eliminating toxic foods, drinking pure water and breathing in fresh non polluted air.

Let's look at this from another angle. If you stand back to look at yourself, look at your whole body, you will see your body is really a digestive organ. It takes in food, distributes nutrients throughout the body where it is used by the cells to reproduce. The liver separates the food and sends the valuable nutrients to the cells. The waste material is sent to kidneys and to the bladder. Then the fecal material is sent to the large intestines where it is excreted.

If we eat toxic foods, breathe in toxic fumes and drink water containing toxic chemicals we develop diseases. Then we can conclude the source of living in good health depends upon the type of food we eat, the water we drink and the air we breathe.

There is no one treatment for cancer. Chemotherapy, radiation, and surgery will not cure or prevent cancer. There is no drug, vaccine or therapy that will cure cancer. The only way to prevent cancer from spreading and to delay its reproduction is from proper nutritional planning.

An overweight woman goes to visit her doctor to be treated for a stomachache. The doctor prescribes a pill to ease her pain. Yet he doesn't treat her problem. He doesn't address the real reason for her condition. He fails to treat the whole body. He relies on drugs to remedy the situation. Drugs will not cure her condition. The whole body must be treated and the source can only be through nutrition. Most doctors today advise the person who has cancer to use chemotherapy, radiation and surgery all of which have many side effects. This they call "The Gold Standard" for Cancer.

Years ago Christopher Columbus was jailed because he refuted the gold standard of his day – "The world was flat". He left Italy, backed by the queen and king of Spain, to embark on his ocean voyage to the Americas and the rest is history. There was the bleeding of sickly people in the early years wherein doctors bleed their gouty patients.

They also believed this was the gold standard treatment for gout. Now we know darn well it was the wrong method to perform. Dentist years ago pulled teeth without Novocain because this was the gold standard of the day. Today we know it was cruel and ridiculous.

Over the years we have seen many gold standard treatments to be considered inappropriate and other therapies taking their place. The gold standard treatment today for cancer chemotherapy, radiation and surgery will someday be replaced with alternative therapies as I have outlined in this book. In the not too distant future we will ask why the medical profession ever initiated the treatment of Chemotherapy, Radiation and Surgery as the first line of defense against Cancer. We will look back and say – The use of chemotherapy and radiation was a cruel unjust treatment for the sick. We will wonder why they ever started to administer this type of unscrupulous dangerous treatment.

Additional resources can be obtained from: American Cancer Association. Telephone number 1-800-227-2345.

3 NATURAL ALTERNTIVES FOR TREATMENT OF BREAST CANCER

Aromatase Inhibitors: According to scientists in   Germany at the University of Munster, if one eats aromatase inhibitors these inhibitors will prevent aromatase enzyme from developing phase one cancer in normal cells. Within the normal cells are estrogen receptors (ER) alpha and beta cells. These cells stimulate tissue growth in young women during normal breast development. When the breasts are completely developed, estrogen receptors can continue to bind with the excessive estrogen through aromatization process and can lead to rapid growth and proliferation of mutated breast cells. If this aromatization process is inhibited with aromatase inhibitors the excess estrogen will not spread cancer. Drugs like tamoxifen increase (ER) alpha expression and left (ER) beta unchanged while the aromatase inhibitors up (ER) beta cells and blocked the spreading of Cancer.

We can find aromatase inhibitors in Plants. Nature has given us plant herbs which are much effective than tamoxifen which is used today by doctors to control estrogen overstimulation.

I have listed the powerful plant aromatase inhibitors below which can be a much preferred choice:

- Chrysin

- Quercetin

- Reservatol

- Apigenin

- Genistein

- Oleuropein

These are powerful flavonoids and are found in whole foods. They can also be purchased from online health and vitamin shops and at your local health food stores. As a note, grapefruit should not be eaten because it is involved in breaking down an enzyme P450 which can inhibit sex hormones in the body and is not recommended.

For more information: www.jmbblog.coon/2009/07cancer-alternativetreatments-digest-part-38-natural-arom.3/22/2012

4 END STAGE OF CANCER

After undergoing cancer treatment and being told by oncologists that nothing more can be done for treatment of cancer you will probably come to a conclusion that there isn't very much left to do other than accept and give up desire to live. Well, if a person takes this negative approach to his illness he is lost. When he has surpassed stage four cancer and is in a dilemma, feels mentally and physically exhausted and has no one to turn to, he should review the information on the previous pages. He should pay special attention to the topics; changing diet, staying away from cancer producing foods, taking on a positive attitude, practicing meditation, giving off good vibrations to others, and reflecting on an overall feeling of being cured.

Feed the mind good thoughts, believe you will be healed and maybe physiologically you may be healed. Follow through in making this happen.

We all have cancer cells in our body, some lay dormant some spread quickly depending on how we keep our immune systems working. Remember, not all cancer patients follow a straight and narrow path when suffering from cancer. All persons are different and cancer cells work differently with each person.

Cancer cells might spread to just a few areas of the body. Then it is possible cancer cells might lay dormant and then a cancer person   may be free from cancer maybe for five to ten years and maybe more. So don't be afraid, your world is not coming to end, take one day at a time. The most common areas where cancer spreads and invades the body is the Liver, Breast, Thyroid. Kidney, Prostate, Lungs. From these organs it spreads to the bones hitting the Spine, Pelvis, Ribs, Skull, and Upper Arms

To learn more about your type of cancer, seek out cancer survivors who have had the same type of cancer and make arrangements to speak to them personally. You might feel much better to hear it from survivors who will give you advice on how to help you ward off the uncertainties as may or may not develop in your case.

Investigate and use the same beliefs they used. Study, do research on your type of cancer, seek and ask questions. We are fortunate in our society to have information available free to us on the internet, from local libraries and local cancer associations.

One may believe that with stage four cancer there isn't much that can be done to prevent cancer from spreading. When a person has stage four cancer the idea of being cared for, washed or fed by another is unpleasant and unnatural. Not only is the idea of dying unspeakable, but to suffer the pains of cancer is unbearable.

Keep a positive attitude, seeking out friends whose positive thoughts can ease your pain and give comfort. This was proven by Dr. Sigmund Freud the psychologist who claimed there is a relationship between mind and body. His research found through patient's feedback, the mind can be subjected into stimulating positive thoughts relating these thoughts to the body(soma).

Through the use of psychotherapy all thoughts and conditions of diseases can be eliminated by training the mind to believe the disease will be cured. If the autonomic system is made to relax and not send signals out to the sympathetic system's nerve endings, the body will not react with stress. The parasympathetic system will take over and calm the body preventing stress from taking over which psychologists believe to be the cause of all disease. All thoughts and conditions of diseases are deriving out of signals from the brain.

Training the mind to become positive, in accepting help from others, giving love, spreading positive thoughts will reverse diseases. This idea initiated by Dr. Sigmund Freud was name Psychology and was developed into Psychotherapy then into Psychoanalysis.

You have probably heard a lot about cancer victims suffering from excruciating pain and fear this the most. We are very fortunate in our day and age we have in our modern day medical arsenal, drugs called opiates that can eliminate pain and make dying peaceful even though they are habit forming. If it's an unpleasant feeling having someone treat you like an invalid, this can be remedied with learning to shake off bad

feelings and take on positive feelings. Speak to others who have the same disease. You might be happy to learn how they survived.

CANCER PRODUCING ADDITIVES-BANNED COLOR ADDITIVES

- Butter Yellow-Green1
- Green 2, Green 3, Yellow 3,4
- Red 1,2,4,32
- Sudan
- Violet 1
- Cinamyl Anthuvanlate
- Cobalt Salts
- Coumarin
- Cyclamate
- Dethyl Procarbonate
- Ethlyene Glycol
- Monochloracidic Acid
- Nordihyudroqualacetic Acid
- Oil of Calamus
- Polyoxyethylene Sterate
- Myr 45
- Safrole
- Thiourea

ATTACH THIS LIST TO YOUR REFRIGERATOR AND REFER TO THIS LIST FROM TIME TO TIME. (Complements of: CARE FOR THE LIVING)

5 AHCC

AHCC (Active hexose correlated compound) is made up of extracts of several types of mushrooms. These mushrooms have been found to be an excellent source of nourishment to stimulate the (NK) normal killer cells to attack cancer cells within our body, in so doing destroying cancer cells. The action of AHCC is to build up the immune system preventing good cells to die, and preventing cancer cells to metastasize.

Conventional medicine has over the years frowned upon other means of treating cancer and have stuck to treating cancer patients with only one final procedure in using Chemotherapy and Radiation and Surgery. If this doesn't control or eradicate cancer then they refer the cancer patient to Hospice.

It is well known that Japanese have been consuming Shitake mushrooms for many years and have lived well beyond the age of one hundred. In Japan AHCC is prescribed by physicians and the results when combined with a hybrid mushroom has proven potent as one of the world's most powerful and safe simulators of the immune system. AHCC is well absorbed in the stomach and improves the immune system.

Here are some ways in which AHCC boosts the immune system:

1. It increases the explosive granules with the   NK cells.
2. It stimulates cytokines production which acts to stimulate immune function.
3. Increased numbers of lymphocytes increasing T cells.
4. Increase level of interferon which inhibits replication of viruses.
5. Stimulates the production of TNF proteins that help to destroy cancer cells.

According to the clinical trial published in the International Journal of Immunotherapy, AHCC lowers the tumor makers (material that detects the presence of tumors) found in patients with ovarian, prostate, breast and other cancers. It has been shown to prevent the recurrence of liver cancer.

Product can be ordered under the name of ImmPower @ American BioSsciences Inc: Telephone: 845-727-0800.

Information regarding AHCC can be obtained from (HIS) Health Sciences Institute.com or by calling: 800-981-7157

6 PHOTOLUMINESCENSE

Photo stands for light and luminescence stands for emission of light. What does this process do? It kills cancer cells within the blood. How? By passing ultra violet light rays over blood which is withdrawn from the cancer patient. The theory was popular in the 1930s and was pushed aside since the discovery of antibiotics.

Today due to the dangerous resistant antibiotics the practice of PT (photoluminescence) is now being practiced by many doctors. The procedure is simple. The patient's blood is withdrawn from a vein and passed through a machine which irradiates the blood with ultra violet light rays and then the blood is sent back into the vein. In so doing the blood is oxygenated and kills cancer cells without harming the good cells.

The process was first discovered by Dr. Emmett K. Knott who irradiated the blood of humans back in the 1928. By 1934 Dr. Knott and Dr. Virgil K. Hancock published their paper on Photo therapy. The process of PT has no known side effects. The doctors practiced 300,000 tests which shows PT to work in the treatment of cancer, viral infections, AIDS, Osteomyelitis,

Septicemia, Virolent infections of the blood, Emphysema, Fibrosis and immune deficiency problems. The FDA has approved a new PL machine invented by Johnson and Johnson with Dr. Elderson. The machine is called "Extracorporeal Photopheresis Blood Irradiator"

A good source of additional information can be found on the web:

www.mindwelldir.org/docsd/uvlight/uvlight3.htm

The book "Into the Light", written by Dr. William Campbell Douglass is a good additional source of information.

Here are some of the doctors who perform ultraviolet Blood Irradiation:

Arizona: Dr. Frank W. George, 12611 N. 103rd Ave, Suite A, Sun City, AZ AZ99503

California: Dr. Robert Rown, Trinity Health Club, 2200 Clounty Center Dr. H Santa Rosa, CA 95403

Colorado: Dr. Thomas R. Lawrence, DC Alternate Medical Center of Colorado, PC 801 Youngfield St 8117, Golden, CO 80401

Florida: Dr. Martin Dayton DO, 1860 Collins Avenue, Sunny Isles Beach, FL433160

Massachusetts: Dr. Ruben Oganesov, Allston Physical Medicine Center, 39 Righton Avenue Allston, MA 02234

New Jersey: Dr. Ivan Kroh, Longivity Medical LLC, 540 Bordentown Ave, South Amboy, NJ

New York: Dr. Steven Bock, M.D. Hinebock Health Center, 108 Montgomery Street, Rhinebock, 12572

Pennsylvania: Dr.William Glen Kracht, Woodlands Healing Research Center, 5724 Clymer Rd, Quakertown, PA 1895

Here is a therapy which has been suppressed and kept hidden from the public for many years. What is FSM? It is called (Frequency Specificmicrocurrent). It was used many years ago and discovered by Dr. Royal Rife in the 1930s.

The machine was not very well received by the medical profession or by the FDA (Food & Drug Admin) which in turn took immediate action to condemn the Rife machine and ordered the machine taken off the market and warned doctors their licenses would be revoked if anyone was caught using such a machine.

Over the years the machine was put aside until Dr. James Barre improved on the machine and received backing from his peers, developing the machine under the name of Rife/Barre.

The action of the machine works whereby tiny electrodes are connected to the injured area or tissue and an electrical current is passed into the area which causes the cells to resonate. All cells resonate at certain frequencies and when

they are stimulated to a certain frequency they increase their production of ATP (energy molecules). Research in the field of electromagnetic energy has shown FSM increases the action of protein synthesis by 20%. It helps to rebuild damaged tissues and FSM helps to build parts of the body, tissues, ligaments and organs.

Researchers have also found EM (energy magnetic field) causing tumors to regress and create immunity to cancer. Today there has been new studies on the use of the Rife/Barre machine and many confirm it to be useful in treating all sorts of life threatening diseases.

If more information is needed internet search on the following subjects:

FDA: Paper on pulsated, electric field, RF Bio effects. Videos are also available: go to: Rife/Barre. You can contact Nature's Way at 2246 Citrus Blvd #393, Leesburg, FL 24748, Tel: 888-563-5335

In 1980 Dr. Abulkaiam Shamsuddin at the University of Maryland pioneered research of IP6 which is also known as inositol hexophosphate or phytic acid. Research has shown it to be astounding as an alternative in the treatment and prevention of Cancer. IP6 is one of the B vitamins and has been proven to change cancer cells physiology by normalizing the sugar production of cancerous cells altering their gene expression toward healthful conditions.

IP6 protects against Cancer in many ways. It normalizes the rate of cell growth, helps to normalize cell physiology, enhances (NK) white blood cells, inhibits inflammation, exhibits potent antioxidant activity, affects angiogenesis (inhibits the formation of new blood vessels), and inhibits metastasis (the spread of cancer cells throughout the body).

IP6 has been tried in the treatment of prostate cancers, Gastric cancers, Glioiblastoma (brain tumors) and ongoing research has found it to be also useful in the possible treatment of diabetes, depression, osteoporosis, heart disease and kidney stones.

There are some naturopath doctors and other unorthodox doctors who are recommending IP6 in conjunction with modern "gold standard" treatment for the prevention and treatment of cancer. This can be highly useful to anyone who is of high risk, who has had a recurrence of cancer or is looking to prevent cancer. I strongly believe this treatment is presently being considered by traditional doctors who are using it as part of their protocol.

IP6 is supplied in capsule and powder form and can be purchased from:Vitacost.com More information can be obtained online at: www.IP6.com

9 INSULIN POTENTIATION THERAPY

Insulin potentiation therapy IPT was discovered in 1930 by a Dr. Perez's grandfather in Mexico City. In 1950 he transferred the study to his son. It was a study done in the treatment cancer patients of which the study was shown to be greatly successful. Some doctors believe it is just another money making scheme practiced by quack doctors whose only desire is to shake down prospective willing patients who will try anything to alleviate their physical and mental pain.

I had a friend whose mother was suffering from bladder Cancer and was being treated at one of the biggest hospitals in the East. After the treatment of the standard protocol - Chemotherapy, Radiation and Surgery she was told there wasn't anything more that could be done for her.

They recommended Hospice a place where they would assist her with pain medication and make it much more comfortable as she approached the end.

I took it upon myself to do a little research regarding her situation. I searched the internet and came across Dr. Linchitz located in Long Island, NY. He learned he had lung Cancer and went along with the oncologist's suggestion to undergo the standard treatment options. His lung was removed and he was told that the Cancer was fully removed. Six months later he was told the cancer had spread and the other lung would need to be treated. He refused and investigated alternative ways to cure cancer. He came across IPT, Insulin Potentiation Therapy which he used on himself and eventually cured his own cancer. I questioned this and wondered whether it would be a therapy I could recommend to my friend for his mother. I telephoned Dr. Linchitz' office and wanted to know how long after his treatment had the doctor remained Cancer free?

The reply was ten years to the present. I asked if maybe this therapy could be applied to bladder cancer patients and the answer was "Yes". I also wanted to know if vitamins are administered along with the IPT treatment and the answer was "Yes". If you know anyone who is in the same position as my friend, by all means don't wait. This treatment in my estimation is a very viable and successful one.

If you are a diabetic however, consult with your primary doctor to see if IPT is right for you. If not then ask your doctor to look into the other therapies listed on previous pages of this book. Cancer cells have an affinity for glucose which is food that fuels them. They need glucose to multiply. Cancer cells have a great number of insulin receptors within their cells, thereby causing normal cells to divide and turn into cancer cells. When insulin is injected in the patient's blood, the cancer cell absorbs the insulin first cutting out the normal cells which do not have a great number of cancer receptors.

A few minutes later the chemo drug methotrexate, in low doses is administered (injected) into the patient's blood and the cancer cells die. The good part, is only small amounts of the chemo drug is administered reducing nausea and dangerous side effects. There have been only a few doctors who practice this therapy in the US. This therapy does not need approval by the FDA for it has been practiced over seventy years.

If a patient has been told they are in stage four of Cancer, they have alternative therapies to choose. I believe IPT is a good therapy to use along with the present day chemotherapy drugs. What we are chiefly concerned with is the patient and his or her cure. The final choice is left with the patient. You are given only one body, take care of it. Following is a good reference for a better understanding of the IPT website:
www.Linchitzmedicalwellness.com

Here you will be able to see a video of Dr. Linchitz explaining IPT and how it helped him to stop the spread of his lung cancer. You can also contact his office at: 516-759-4200.

10 OZONE

When a molecule of oxygen is oxidized to a third atom of oxygen it becomes ozone (03). Ozone is found in the atmosphere as a blue color and has a somewhat fresh odor that turns the sky blue. It has been named ozien (to smell) by the Greeks. It comes in second to Fluorine as a disinfectant, oxidizer, detoxifiers and deodorizer. Some alternative cancer doctors are using O3 in conjunction with the administration of other alternative therapies such as IPT (Insulin Potentiation Therapy) to treat stage four cancers. Cancer cells survive and multiply easy and fast without oxygen. When there is an abundance of oxygen cancer cells die. They are anaerobic in nature - meaning without oxygen.

Normal cells require oxygen to multiply (aerobic) – meaning with oxygen. When O3 is injected into the blood of the patient it enters the blood vessels and combines with the proteins, carbohydrates and fatty acids. As it flows into the blood vessels it decomposes into H2O2 (hydrogen peroxide) which in turn penetrates the red blood vessels. Nitrous Oxide (NO) is formed which dilates the blood vessels and improves oxygen flow. Cancer cells do not like oxygen. The more oxygen that is admitted into the blood vessels the less likely the cancer cells will survive in an oxygen concentration.

Additional information can be found on the following website:

www.promolifehealth.com/about-ozone-information/whatisozone-therapy.

11 FLAXSEED OIL THERAPY

Dr. Johanna Budwig a leading authority on the use of flaxseed oil considers unsaturated fats, specifically, Flaxseed oil, to be an important fat in the control of Arthritis, Heart Infractions, Cancer and other diseases.

She postulates sun rays give off negative electrons and photons which move and cause a magnetic field. These rays which shine upon plants cause the process of photosynthesis which helps the plant cells to multiply. In humans this is also true; sunlight rays stimulate the production of new cells and keep the body in good shape. The use of saturated fats in humans interferes with the electrons being transferred into the body cells and thereby prevents replication of cells. Unsaturated fats such as Flaxseed oil along with no salt cottage cheese produce electrons which are attracted to the photons of the sun's rays.

Thus flaxseed oil along with proper nutrients stimulates healthy cell division and cures the above mentioned diseases. Dr. Budwig stated in one of her speeches that "In a patient who was sick, doctors said the patient didn't have more than an hour or two to live, and patient was moribund (in a dying state, they gave the patient simple natural foods(which includes the unsaturated fat,- Flaxseed oil, the patient survived."

The electrons found in unsaturated fats such as flaxseed oil have the same wavelength as sunlight. When we eat these fats electrons are distributed to all other organs of the body. The immune system, the endocrine system and the reproductive system all aide in the oxygenation of the blood.

Man has a true relationship with the sun's wave length photons. By consuming these electron healthy foods, we can deduce life can be disease free and those strands of DNA which are attached to our chromosomes, telomeres will not be compromised and life can be extended beyond belief.

A quote from Doctor Budwig follows:

"Flax oil is a cure aide against arthritis, heart infarction, cancer and other diseases. We have to see that radiation treatment and operations are regarded as obsolete in our era. We do not find these methods convincing and there is not one scientific argument which justifies the use of this kind of un-biological radiation".

Keep this statement in mind if you are ever considering radiation surgery.

Additional References follow:

1. Flax oil As A True Aid Against Arthritis, Heart Infarction, Cancer And Other Diseases. Published by: Apple publishing 1994

2. Dr. Johanna Budwig's, "The Oil Protein Diet."
   Apple Publishing Company, www.apple publishing.com

Where to Buy Flaxseed Oil:Barleans Organic Oils, 4936 Lake Terrell Road, Ferndale.Washington,98248

12 VENUS FLY TRAP

Venus Fly Trap has an extract called "Carnivora" which can digest and kill insects. It is amazing how this plant does not have a digestive system but it has unique active constituents Quercetin and Muricetin, both strong bioflavonoids. These bioflavonoids break down protein making it digestible to the Venus Fly Trap plant.

I was always intrigued with the amazing way in which the Venus Fly Trap swallows the fly and how on the very next day when I re-examined the plant the fly was completely digested.

In the early 1970s, a German physician Helmut Keeler marveled at how the Venus fly trap digested proteins without a digestive system. He also understood that cancer cells actually leak out proteins. He concluded if these cancer cells can leak out proteins maybe the Venus Fly Trap extract can kill them without harming normal cells. Dr Keeler believed the compounds found in the Venus Fly Trap such as, droserone(D) plumbagin(P) and hydroplumbagin(HP) are oxidation catalysts found in other carnivorous plants.

Carnivora which has been used to treat various conditions of blood diseases, inflammation, immune stimulation, improves general all around health. Some scientists and researchers have reported that they have had   significant response rate in advance cancers, chronic fatigue, Lyme disease, parasites, and inflammatory bowel conditions and other major diseases.

In Germany an extract of Carnivora is used in the treatment of chronic diseases in most forms of cancer, colitis, multiple sclerosis, all types of herpes chronic arthritis, and almost any immune deficiency such as AIDS .

You can purchase the herb known as Carnivora in the United States. It can be administered as an extract and in a capsule form, orally or by injections or inhalation. The product has been used legally in the United States.

For more information go to:

www.CarnivoraResearchInternation.com.

13 CATS CLAW

It seems this is a funny name for an herb, but it has been used for more than 100 years, here in America and in Europe. As a young boy working in my father's drug store dusting the old bottles of herbs, I came across the label Cat's Claw. I remembered the name of the herb but I didn't know what it was used for. After doing a little research I found Cat's Claw is being used today in the treatment of Cancer.

Cancer researchers are finding Cat`s claw beneficial in stimulating the immune system, preventing inflammation and increasing white blood cells. In 1989 a Australian doctor isolated six alkaloids from the root of Cats Claw known as Uncaria tomentosa. Of these six alkaloids four have an affinity to enhance the production of phagocytes, stimulating the macrophage to engulf, digest harmful organisms, within

the blood. Cat`s Claw has been beneficial in the treatment of cancer, arthritis, bursitis, genital herpes, herpes zoster, all allergies, systemic maladies, environmental toxic poisoning, and numerous other diseases . It has been found to out surpass the traditional herbs golden seal, Echinacea, Maitake, Shiitake Mushrooms, Ginseng, Astrgaalus and other natural herbs.

Buy from: Penn Herb Co: 800-523-9971

14 AVEMAR

It was Dr. Albert Szent-Gyuorgyia a Noble Prize recipient who in 1937 started his research into wheat germ called DMVQ which he believed would prohibit cancerous cells from growing and multiply throughout the body. In 1989 Dr. Hidvegi of Hungary picked up where Dr. Szent left off and continued to proceed with the production of DMGQ which he named "Avemar" after the Virgin Mary.

Avemar is believed to help prevent nausea and stomach distress while the cancer patient undergoes Chemotherapy and Radiation. It also rejuvenates the immune system by increasing the T-cells and B-cells whereby preventing the recurrence of cancer.

It also speeds cancer cell death by interfering with the absorption of glucose. All good cells and cancer cells have an affinity to absorb glucose yet cancer cells somehow have first choice sucking up glucose which is necessary for the cells to replicate. Avemar has the ability to interfere with cancer cells and reduces glucose production. As a result cancer cells die without any affect upon good cells.

There have been many cancer patients who have undergone Chemotherapy and Radiation and who have taken Avemar along with these treatments and who have successfully reduced their nausea and stomach distress. Avemar should be the choice. Avemar is a wheat germ extract and there can be side effects. If one is allergic to wheat and gluten consult with your physician before taking Avemar.

Avemar can be obtained from:

The American Bioscience Company Tel#: 845-727-0800

15 DOCTORS DIE FROM OBESITY

I had the occasion to attend a lecture at Yale University one evening. The topic was "Doctors Die Young." This lecture was given by a veterinarian who during his last year of medical school had to write a thesis on why doctors die at an early age. He studied the cadavers of doctors who died over the past years. Much to his chagrin, most of them died due to being overweight with excessive fat accumulated around each   of their internal organs.

The fat surrounded their organs suffocated the heart causing it to stop. This fat accumulation attracts cancer cells and is   a host to them causing them to multiply and metastasize throughout the body.

The average ages these doctors died were 55 and 59 due to the accumulation of excessive fat, lack of proper nutrition, and lack of exercise. They did not believe in vitamins or herbal medication. They followed their own medical knowledge treating themselves with drugs, instead of following a nutritional protocol.

When a patient visits a doctor, in many cases doctors don`t have time to go over the patent's nutrition, ask about his health, the type of workplace, the patient's home life or the patient's diet. The doctor treats the ailment. If the patient has a pain in the head he prescribes pain pills.

If the patient has a stomachache, he prescribes stomach antacids, and so forth, never trying to get at the source of the ailment. The doctor issues a prescription and sends the patient home to continue to eat the same fat foods and has the patient return if the symptoms do not subside. The vicious cycle of treatment continues week after week, month after month, trying one drug after another and referral to other specialists who also join in the vicious cycle to remedy the patient's problem.

The doctors should consider examining the patient as a whole person, study his nutritional habits, what he eats, what kind of pressure he is facing daily and other personal problems he is experiencing in his daily life. Today, some medical schools are including in their curriculum bedside manners and nutritional courses so that the physicians can become better acquainted with the patient.

I believe if the doctors who die so young kept themselves on a low fat diet, followed a good nutritional diet, taking vitamins minerals and amino acids, stayed with an all green vegetable diet and eliminated toxic chemicals from their food, they may have lived a much longer life.

16 QUACKWATCH.COM

If after reading the previous pages, you are wondering whether or not to use any of the therapies suggested, click onto Quackwatch.com. Here you will find Quack watch is strongly disfavors use of any therapies and vitamins. This website is against the use of Vitamin C for the treatment of Cancer and disagrees with Dr. Linus Pauling's research on Vitamin C in the treatment of cancer, and the curing of the common cold.

Let's look into the background of the founder of "Quack Watch" – Stephen Barrett, M.D. He graduated from Boston University in 1987 with a degree in internal medicine. He has more than 25 years in this practice.

But I couldn't find any information as to his being a nutritionist. He says, "Vitamin C is worthless in the use of curing the common cold and doesn't do much for all herbs and vitamins. They should be considered unreliable   and in a form of misinformation (quackery)"

What is Quackwatch? It is a non profitable organization with an international network of people who are concerned with health related frauds, myths, fads and fallacies. Are they concerned with the big pharmaceutical companies who have manufactured drugs which are detrimental to the general public and over the years have produced toxic drugs, and have killed over thousands of lives? Are they concerned with the tobacco industry which is   fraudulently selling tobacco products which have been known to kill many Americans and Europeans?

Are they also concerned with the big alcohol manufacturers, who through false advertising state, "Alcohol prevents hardening of the arteries."? Many Americans who become alcoholic die of cirrhosis of the liver, and kidney failure.

Are they concerned with Coffee a multi- million-dollar industry which publicizes, "Coffee is good for the body, and good in preventing heart trouble"? When so many Americans consume so much Caffeine which is a drug found in Coffee, it a can cause myocardial infraction, leading to death.

Are they concerned with Sugar, also a multibillion dollar product? The big manufacturers state, "Eating dark chocolate is great for the brain and for your cholesterol, helps clean your arteries and keeps them free from the accumulation of lipids(fats)." When today there is an epidemic of obesity in America. Sugar producing manufacturers, including drug companies who over the years have fraudulently, with intent to earn big bucks, undergone the most paramount health related frauds we know of today.

They are given a slap on the wrist and fined billions yet they are not closed down and are permitted by the FDA to resume operating. The FDA states "We can`t closed these big pharmaceutical companies down because they would put a lot of people out of work and add them to the unemployment role.

Quackwatch is definitely looking the other way and is not living up to their original nonprofit organization Bylaws, which state, "Their aim and purpose of establishing their organization is to investigate health related fraudulent matters."

Remember be careful when making a judgment or reaching a decision. When searching Quackwatch it might prejudicial and hearsay. Confirm what you have read then make your decision. GOOD LUCK.

17 OBESITY

Obesity is another topic which is important if one desires to live for a long time. If you have tried drugs to lose weight you are going in the wrong direction. No matter what drugs or herbs or fruits or vinegars are tried, losing weight is a waste of time and money. The average American is between thirty to forty pounds overweight. Perhaps by the time this book is published that number may grow to between forty to sixty pounds. Three out every five persons are considered overweight and obesity has been classified as epidemic in America.

I have listed below topics which are considered beneficial and important if you are trying to lose weight.

1. Readjusting your food intake and changing eating habits

2. Choosing the right food

3. Balancing Acid and Alkaline Foods

4. Exercising

5. Fasting

6. Detoxification

7. Meditation

8. Positive Attitude

Choosing the right food is important - eating fewer carbohydrates and replacing them with more protein, fresh fruits and vegetables. There are two types of foods – macronutrients, which are carbohydrates, protein and fats. The other type is micronutrients - vitamins and minerals, which are found in fruits and vegetables. Replacing macronutrients with micronutrients foods are considered a better choice. Balance food intake with more alkaline foods - vegetables, sprouts, fruits, sprouted breads, sprouted wraps and gluten yeast free breads. Oils- Olive, Coconut. Flaxseed and Avocado. Also add pecans, pistachios, prunes and hazelnuts.

Exercise forty minutes a day, walking or working in a garden would do fine - leaving the TV and the Computer for a time. This will stimulate the blood flow throughout your body and will prevent your muscles from becoming atrophic (stiff-immobile.)

Practicing fasting one day a week will definitely alleviate your pain in many areas of the body. Pain from arthritis, rheumatoid arthritis, stomach gastritis will be reduced by practicing fasting.

Blood pressure will be reduced along with a low diabetic reading and with a lighter feeling throughout the body. Fasting has been practiced in India and China for centuries and has been shown to keep weight down. This is a method you can also use in order to lose weight without the use of toxic medications.

Detoxification is another method which stimulates peristalsis in the large intestine and causes evacuation of digestive foods from the rectum. Various herbal drugs can be used to clean out the digestive tract like senna leaves and soluble and non-soluble fibers. Castor oil was used forty years ago and some doctors still recommend this oil to pregnant women before child birth to reduce the large intestine so the new born can evacuate the uterus with less restriction. Over the counter preparations that also can be used are fleet enemas, methylcellulose powder, Metamucil and citrate of magnesia.

Meditation, a practice commonly used by in Asia has been used for well over one hundred years to improve the mind,

relax the body and give one a sense of wellbeing - a relationship with the power and spiritual touch with the force of the universe and God. Some religious persons recite the rosary as a source of meditating, forgetting all thoughts, concentrating on the beads as their recite the prayers daily.

Positive attitudes are also important when starting a reducing diet. A positive attitude will help you to manage and continue with the demands of restricting your special habitual foods. Stay away from negative people who only will bring you down on your practice. Rely only on yourself continuing to think positive. By reducing your daily food intake, selecting the right foods and eliminating carbohydrates, staying with vegetables, fruits and micronutrients your weight will begin to reduce and in no time at all you will reach your goal losing weight.

I would like to paint you a scenario. Let`s sit back and relax and visualize a private island somewhere in the Pacific without any persons living on this island. An obese three hundred pound American middle aged man is left alone on this island with only

the food on the island – fruits, pure fresh water, fish and vegetables.

After a year he returns home. Would he have lost weight? You bet! But after being back for a time, does he put on more weight? Of course. Why? Because he is back macronutrients – carbohydrates, fats, sugars, and his old diet. He is putting on more weight than he had before he went on this trip. What does this prove? It proves you can lose weight if you eat less and only the foods which are classified as micronutrients.

REMEMBER: THE LESS YOU EAT THE LONGER YOU LIVE.

LET FOOD BE YOUR MEDICINE

18 THE BRAIN

I would like to compare the automobile's battery to the human brain. The battery controls the electrical system of the auto by sending out electricity to all the parts of the motor. If the battery has a crack in it, or it leaks acid or it has suffered a blow from a car accident, the battery does not function properly and the car sends out irregular movements and sometimes dies out.

Likewise, the human brain sends out electrical stimuli to the five senses of the body - Sight, Hearing, Tasting, Smell and Touch. There are also other stimuli beyond the five senses and they are - Temperature, Kinesthetic Sense, Pain Sense, Balance Sense and Accelerated senses.

The brain is divided into three hemispheres- the Forebrain, the Midbrain and the Hindbrain. The Forebrain consists of the Cerebrum, Amygdala, and the Hippocampus. The Midbrain, consists of the Tectum and the Tegmentum, sometimes they are mentioned together with the Hindbrain, Cerebellum, Pons, and the Medulla Obligata.

The Hypothalamus is the section that controls memory and is considered an important section of the brain. When a stimulus is sent out to the hypothalamus it sends neuron signals to the pituitary gland and from there the pituitary gland sends out signals to other parts of the brain. If areas of the brain are destroyed or suffer a blow through an accident, neurons do not function properly and the body suffers all sorts of inactions. Therefore, we can see the similarity between the car battery and the brain.

When a stressful condition arises with the body, stimuli activate the three communication systems which are: The Voluntary Nervous System that sends messages to the muscles, the

Autonomic Nervous System which consists of the Sympathetic and Parasympathetic system. The Sympathetic Nervous System controls the emergency system and gets us up to run, secreting the hormone epinephrine (adrenaline). The Parasympathetic Nervous System controls the quieting down and calming effect secreting the hormone cortisol. The third system is the Neuroendocrine System, which controls the metabolic and sex function.

You may ask what the brain has to do with extending life. If the brain controls all the actions of the body and can disable movement and prevent cells from excreting dopamine and other hormones, then scientists can stimulate sections of the brain to extend the waste products of the DNA Telomeres and prevent aging. The early Egyptian's, during the procedure of embalming, sucked out the brain of the Pharos through the nostrils believing the brain stored all life's experiences and spiritual beliefs.

How important is the spinal column in the animal kingdom? Here is an example of how the animals search out and consume their prey. It has been known in the animal kingdom, the lion knows from instinct that by biting the spinal column of his prey, it will paralyze the prey's entire body. As the lion approaches his prey it attacks the hind leg and once bitten the prey fails to the ground. Quickly the lion jumps onto its back and bites the neck.

This causes paralysis to the animal attacked. The lion along with other lions in the pride eat the animal alive. Remarkable indeed. Today, doctors are practicing acupuncture which is a practice of sticking needles into the various locations of the body to intercept the electric current supplied by the various systems of the brain. By doing so they can eliminate pain, stop headaches, relieve leg cramps, and stop free radicals from developing.

They believe cutting off nerves to the various parts of the body can stop pain. In some cases this procedure can be helpful, in others not so helpful.

We see how important the brain is in controlling all bodily activities. How manipulating certain sections of the brain can trigger either a positive or a negative response. The study of the brain is in its infancy, and the scientists of tomorrow will spend more time trying to expand knowledge of the brain, how it works and how it can cure diseases in patients with neurological disorders and someday maybe even extend life forever.

19 THE IMMUNE SYSTEM

The immune system defends the body from foreign invaders such as viruses and bacteria. It is the second line of defense which includes the lymphatic system. This lymphatic system regulates the flow of liquid throughout the circulatory system. There are over 100 lymph nodes throughout the body and when there is an infection within the body, these lymph nodes become inflamed and cause diseases. The immune system cells are white blood cells which come to the aid of the cells when there is an infection in the body. They are called lymphocytes. There are two kinds of lymphocytes - T- cells and B- cells. T- cell receptors interact with the MHC molecules which are on most cells and help T- cells recognize antigen fragments along with the B- cells known for the production of antibodies to fight off foreign invaders.

T-cells are made from the thymus gland and B- cells are derived from the bone marrow. We can see the glands which are important to protect the immune system are the Thymus gland the Spleen, Bone marrow and Liver.

The Thymus gland is located wrapped around the thyroid gland in the neck area. It is important because it can produce T-cells which can fight off the foreign invaders of the lymphatic system; keeping the immune system healthy. The Spleen which is situated below the left lobe of the liver and adjacent to the pancreas, very close to the small intestine, is also important for the production of antibodies. These antibodies launch onto antigens for the destruction by other immune system cells.

Macrophages and Neutrophils circulate in the blood and survey the body for foreign substances when they find these substances they act upon them and kill them. Yet sometimes the surrounding tissues become inflamed and various diseases can develop. We can see that the phagocytes and the macrophages and the NK cells can help with the eradication of foreign invaders in our blood and protect us from diseases of all kind. Yet we must be vigilant with building our immune system and learn all we can in order to survive.

Following are the leading contributing factors that can cause decreased immune system functionality:

1. Radiation, Chemotherapy

2. Surgery

3. Anti-Inflammatory

4. Lack of Sleep

5. Stress

6. Depression

7. Air, water and soil pollution

8. Vitamin deficiency

9. Improper diet

20 BUILDING OUR IMMUNE SYSTEM

If you are wondering how we can prevent the immune system from breaking down and causing maladies in the body, we can start with the following: faulty meal planning, an acidic environment, lack of proper sleep nutrients, vitamins, amino acids and minerals, overwork, and excessive stress in our everyday life. We lose are ability to concentrate and lose strength which can effect emotional and physiological factors. This can create a domino effect upon all the other organs in our body – the liver, kidney, heart and blood flow are all affected.

The immune suppressors can reduce the reproduction of cells and can in time, if not corrected, stimulate the sudden growth of cancer cells.

I have listed below some immune system suppressors. Look them over and commit them to memory in order to help understand the causes of immune system failure and ultimately how you can help to improve your immune system.

IMMUNE SYSTEM SUPPRESSORS

- Aging
- Allergies
- Pollen
- Drugs
- Viruses and Bacteria
- Yeast, Fungus
- Eliminate Teflon cookware
- Eliminate microwave use
- Toxic chemical

21 IMMUNE SYSTEM SUPPORTERS

On the other side of the spectrum we can increase the basic care of our immune system by considering supporters of the immune system. Our immune system is at its highest when we supply the necessary nutrients, follow a planned diet, eliminate stress in our everyday life and take on a positive attitude. The selecting of immune supporters can be beneficial to persons who are depressed, who suffer from viral and bacterial infections and whose immune system has been compromised by disease especially cancer.

Tests which can determine whether your immune level is normal can be obtained by receiving a CBC; a complete blood test. This test can provide absolute levels of Tm, Ts and B cells and natural killer cells in determining the level of the immune system.

Preventive care is important in one's lifestyle. Good organic food, less stress, exercise, meditation, diet and supplements is the key to better health and the reduction of diseases. Therapies such as FSM (Frequency specific modulation) also Photoluminescence, Insulin Potentiation Therapy (IPT), Ozone (O3) and the oral administration of Avemar, Shitake mushrooms, Carnivora are the main effective remedies to control and keep the immune system functioning on all cylinders. This may contribute to extending the telomeres and in doing so may extend human life.

IMMUNE SYSTEM SUPPORTERS

- Rotating diet
- Choice of Alkaline foods
- Vitamins A, B, C, D, E
- B complex, B12 Metylcobalamine
- Amino acids
- Low fat diet, no sugar
- Caffeine free diet
- Filtered water
- Organic food choices
- Fasting
- No Alcohol
- No tobacco
- Stress free life
- Meditate
- Positive thoughts and outlook
- Essential fatty acids
- Digestive enzymes
- Detoxification
- Fiber, soluble and insoluble.
- Chemical free diet
- Chemical free food
- Organic milk

22 FOOD-BALANCING ACID/ALKALINE FOODS

We have learned in the previous pages, how Cancer develops and survives. We have learned Cancer cells love an acid environment and dislike Oxygen. Therefore, we must concern ourselves with these two factors which if one can prevent these factors from developing cancers we have a good chance in stopping the spread of Cancer.

Foods are classified into basically two categories - Acid and Alkaline. They can be either Acidic or Alkaline. It has investigated by leading researchers; too much acidic food consumed will throw off the balance in our body and make it ideal for cancer cells to multiply. Normal blood has been found to have a ph. of 7.4 chiefly alkaline when it goes lower it becomes acidic in such a medium. The accumulating excessive acid foods in our diet throws off the metabolism of the blood and tissues causing the surrounding normal cells to become cancerous subdivide and survive. It is advisable to try and keep the blood more alkaline by eating alkaline foods and in this way prevent cancer cells form proliferating. A ph range of 6-7.4 is the normal blood range

Listed below is a list of Acidic and Basic Foods.

<u>ACIDIC FOODS</u>:

- Dairy and Eggs
- All soda and diet soda
- All sweeteners
- Flavored water
- Oils
- Milk
- Cooking oils
- Tap water
- Palm oil
- Cotton seed oil
- Sports drinks
- Regular and decaffeinated coffee
- All nuts and seeds:
  - Pecans
  - Pistachios
  - Hazelnuts
- Prunes
- Mayonnaise
- Mustard
- Ketchup
- Pickles
- Vinegar

ALKALINE FOODS

- All Vinegars
- Sprouts
- Fruits
- Breads
- Sprouted breads
- Sprouted wraps
- Gluten yeast free breads

- OILS:
    - Olive
    - Coconut
    - Flaxseed
    - Avocado

23 FIBER

Most everyone owns an automobile and takes good care of its operation. They try to put in the best gas, and have the engine checked annually in order for it to last a long time. The radiator is flushed out cleaned and replaced with new antifreeze. When it comes to cleaning out the digestive system, however many believe it will just take care of itself over time. It seems the caring and attention of the automobile's condition is far more important than maintaining one's own body. Fiber is the main ingredient necessary for flushing out the digestive system.

We can eliminate many common diseases by cleansing the internal organs of the body by using soluble and insoluble foods. Those soluble foods are as follows: oranges, pears, carrots, potatoes, squash oats and barley. The soluble fibers absorb water from the large intestines and in doing so it also sucks out the cholesterol. It also forms a small amount of bulk which is good for the peristalsis

to occur. You can find additional fibers in vegetables, fruits and oat brans. The insoluble fibers form bulk and keeps the intestines open, preventing any cancer cells from forming between the two sides of the intestines. It also causes the bowels to move out the digested food quickly .This fiber has been suggested to cancer patients who have had intestinal cancer. They want the intestinal wall to be free of fecal matter as soon as possible, to get it out of the bowls. In doing so, the bacteria will not accumulate into the walls of the intestine and become a condition known as, DIVERTICULOSIS.

The human body is a very special organism and its digestive system must be in balance. When a limited amount of food is ingested the large intestines do not enlarge and the interior curvature walls adhere to each other.

With this, polyps occur and all sorts of problems arise. If we can eat a well-balanced diet and ingest fiber regularly we can be assured the walls of the intestines will work efficiently and the intestines will work to prevent disease from occurring in the body.

When adding fiber to your diet, go easy with the amount you use. Too much fiber will probably give you gas and indigestion. Go slow at first then gradually add more until your body gets accustomed to it. When choosing fiber it doesn't make any difference if you take soluble or insoluble fiber, either one will give you the same effect. If you desire to lose weight use soluble fiber. Some good advice is to have soluble fiber before your main meal in order to give you a sense of fullness. This will cause you to eat less and eventually you will lose weight.

Supplementing with foods such as fruits and vegetables can also contribute soluble fiber to your diet. Each fruit color defines different nutrients. We then should mix different color fruits and vegetables in our diet in order to give us a variety of plant nutrients (phytonutrients).

A daily salad with your meals is a good idea. The majority of Europeans who eat the Mediterranean diet, which many nutritionists advocate, consume a great deal of salads with unsaturated dressing such as extra virgin olive oil.

It's so ironic that many persons who own automobiles spend so much time and money on the care of their automobiles. When it comes down to taking care of their own health they assume the body will take care of itself. Once again you have only one body it belongs to you, do not let someone else direct you or force you into making a decision. Your life is your own and you have only one life to live. Whatever decisions you make get all the facts second and get second and third opinions. Look outside the area in which you live and make use of your personal computer.

As a precaution it is not advisable to give small children fiber for their intestines are not mature enough to hold a large quantity of fiber. I believe as they grow older then it would be advisable.

If you do plan to take fiber, take it in the morning on an empty stomach which will give the fiber time to work without mixing it with breakfast. If you develop too much bloating, cut down on the quantity and add additional amounts gradually.

24 COLOSTRUM AS CANCER TREATMENT

You might have heard the word Colostrum. It is the first breast secretion delivered by pregnant women and mammals containing essential nutrients, trypsin and protease inhibitors which protect the immune system. Colostrum has been used by Europeans for more than fifty years and has been shown not to have any side effects. It is all called "Mother's Milk". Researchers have found bovine colostrum is much more effective than mother's milk. It contains more high immune factors than mother's milk.

In Dr. Daniel G. Clark's book "Colostrum, Life's First Food" he states, "Bovine colostrum rebuilds the immune system, destroys viruses, bacterial, and fungi, improves healing of all body tissues, helps lose weight, burns fat, increases bone and lean muscle mass and slows down and even reverses aging".

Colostrum contains immune factors. One factor is called immunoglobulin. This factor neutralizes toxins and microbes within the lymph and circulatory system and kills bacteria. Another factor is: Lactoferrin-which is an antibacterial, an antiviral and anti-inflammatory. It has been shown to treat HIV, Cancer, Cytomegalovirus, chronic fatigue, herpes, Candida albicans and other infections caused by bacteria. Lastly it also contains (PRP) proline rich polypeptides. This is a hormone which regulates the thymus gland regulating an overactive immune system.

Colostrum also contains a growth factor called platelet derived growth factor (PDGF), an Insulin like growth factor, transforming growth factors A&B. Epithelial growth factor, and fibroblast growth factors.

Newborn babies have a weak immune system and are in need of colostrum. Today many pediatricians recommend mothers to breast feed their newborn simply due to immune system factors. This is considered a natural food without any toxic effects to the human body.

Remember, any therapy or any product recommended will not cure Cancer but will build your immune system and in so doing will fight off and stimulate macrophages (killer cells) preventing cancer from multiplying. It will slow down the spread of cancer throughout the body.

If you or someone has undergone the conventional treatment for cancer whether it is breast, prostate, bladder or any other cancer and you plan to choose a product that will help to build your immune system, of the two, MCP (modified citrus pectin) and Colostrum, would first start off with Colostrum and them eventually add MCP. Both of these products can be purchased on line or at a health food store. I don't see any reaction if you take these at separate times, one in the morning with meals and one at dinner time followed with a full glass of water. The dosages are on the label of the product.

25 MODIFIED CITRUS PECTIN

Modified Citrus Pectin (MCP), also known as citrus pectin is a form of pectin that has been modified and altered to be much more absorbable to the digestive system. Pectin is a polysaccharide molecule and can found in the citrus fruits such as apples, oranges, peaches and lemons. It is the inner white part of the skin, which contains the pectin. Over the past years MCP has been used as a complementary and alternative cancer therapy and some reports have stated it reduces the spread of prostate, colon, breast, liver and skin cancer.

MCP is also useful in detoxifying heavy metals such as mercury and lead. It has also been reported to reduce tumors strengthening the killing abilities of the Tcells. It prevents the spread of cancer throughout the body and helps to neutralize galexin 3. Galexin 3 is formed by cancer cells and they have a tendency to metastasize (spread throughout the circulatory

system and form tumors). It is also good for patients who have been treated with radiation and chemotherapy and surgery to build the immune system; so as to prevent cancer from reforming. If you or someone you know has undergone the conventional treatment for cancer whether its breast, prostate, bladder or any other cancers and you plan to choose a product to help build your immune system taking MCP and Colostrum is highly recommended.

Toxicity and Side Effects:

MCP can be administered orally in chelating (in getting toxins removed from the blood). There have been no side effects reported but some cases of stomach upset due to the acidity of the pectin have been reported. It can be mixed with food to mask the discomfort of the pectin.

MCP can be purchased at health food stores. More information can be found online: Dr Issac Eliaz website:

www.dreliaz.org/healthreports.com

26 COFFEE

Here is a topic that comes up often and has been somewhat of a controversial subject by many nutritionists and doctors in general. On the plus side, it is well established that coffee both caffeinated and decaffeinated is good for preventing prostate cancer and from hardening of the arteries. It is a substance that will invigorate one's self esteem and gives an early morning lift a get up and go feeling. Taking one a cup of coffee daily can be a blessing in disguise, good for all the senses and gets one awake and stimulated for the day's work. It has also been beneficial for Parkinson's, and Alzheimer's, reducing gallstones and relieving headache pain.

On the other side of the coin we have those health advisors who claim coffee (caffeine) is a habit forming substance. Excess use of caffeine can do just the opposite of the benefits, four cups or more daily of coffee can cause more bodily harm. We have been told coffee is a stimulant and when an excess is consumed it stimulates the heart, can cause myocardial infraction and poor circulation to the chambers of the heart. It can cause headaches, stomach distress, colitis, ulcers, arthritis, osteoarthritis, high blood pressure, and increase cholesterol and triglycerides level in the body. Due to its acidity it can contribute to heart palpitations, bladder and kidney diseases, pancreatic dysfunction and liver diseases.

Pharmacologically caffeine stimulates the symptomatic system which secrets the hormone adrenalin signaling the body to take flight, then the parasymtomatic system, becomes involved and relaxes the body. This is why overdosing of caffeine, excessive consumption of coffee or tea is considered toxic to the body. Protect yourself; stop the excessive consumption of coffee. Be wise, don't compromise your health.

27 VITAMIN C THERAPY

We can add another treatment for cancer, Vitamin C. You can find more than over one thousand web sites for Vitamin C. and how it can prevent cancer. I can give you one type of treatment which is being used today by unorthodox doctors. When using the therapy called Insulin Potentiation Therapy, as outline in the previous pages, Vitamin C is administered with Niacin amide (B3) and other important vitamins along with selenium, Zinc, antioxidants, minerals and enzymes.

Many researchers have concluded Vitamin C in crystalline form as Sodium Ascorbate is less irritating to the stomach. The average dose given is between two and five Gms, daily, taken orally along with B3 500mg tablets. B3 can cause flushing to the face and

when this occurs you are taking too much - reduce the quantity. An overdose of Vitamin C will give you diarrhea. Make sure you cut back on Vitamin C if this occurs. You can add Selenium 600mcg, also Zinc15mg, Calcium 1000mg, Magnesium 500mg, Vitamin A12, 500mcg, Vitamin D3 1000 to 2000 mcg Vitamin B12, 2,000mcg and pancreatic enzymes.

When vitamin C doesn`t work orally, then it can be injected right into the tumor which has been very successful in earlier treatments by many alternative doctors who have used vitamin C in their treatment for tumorous cancers.

There has been reported many uses of vitamin C, besides treating cancers. In Germany, Hungary, and other European countries, Vitamin C has been used for asthma, emphysema, stomach ailments, skin diseases and many more diseases because of its antioxidant properties. There have been no side effects from taking heavy doses of Vitamin C, except cases of diarrhea and stomach cramps.

As people age older one's digestive system doesn't function properly. No matter how much one takes orally it is not absorbed because the intrinsic factor necessary to help digestion is no long active, therefore, Vitamin C must be injected into the blood also with other vitamins if no results are found.

A vitamin C program should be in everyone's protocol whether they are dying of cancer or are just trying to ward off getting cancer. Staying away from saturated fats, eating more plant nutrients and keeping a positive attitude is the best antidote for cancer and all other diseases. A combination of modern medicine with chemotherapy combined with alternative medicine along with the very best of nutrition would be the right path to living a long life.

Whatever therapy is used or is suggested by many researchers, you will find they all include plant nutrients, plenty of fresh fruits, green vegetables, 80% green plant nutrients, with 20% unsaturated fats, along with vitamin supplements and not forgetting Detoxification practices.

Remember food can help cure diseases, but food can also cause diseases. Make sure you select organic, toxic free foods if you intend to live a long time.

More information can be obtained on :

www.Doctoryourself.com-CancerTherapy

I have presented a few therapies on the previous pages which you can review. Take them to your oncologist or primary doctor and ask for feedback. These therapies are good for cancer stages three and four. If you are in this situation and have no other options the try them for what else do you have left? I have read many articles confirming people have been cured from cancer and have lived a normal life with alternative treatments for cancer.

Americans are considered the best fed nation in the world but are considered the least healthy nation in the world. This is because we use a mass amount of insecticides and pesticides over our crops and have adulterated and depleted the soil of its natural minerals and vitamins. Selenium is a chemical which has long been extracted from our soils and is very much needed to counteract cancer cells.

All other antioxidants, Vitamin E, C, D, amino acids, potassium, calcium and a great majority of minerals have also been depleted. Instead, chemicals are absorbed and remain in the soil contaminating the soil for years on end.

We realize insecticides kill insects which are living things. If insecticides can kill insects they can also kill humans. These chemicals lay dormant in the soil and displace worms which are important for soil fertilization. The shredded skin of worms act as fertilizers and worms turn over the soil aerating the soil so plants can be free to absorb moisture and vitamins.

When insects and worms are killed off the whole ecology of nature is upset. This is when food which is grown from these types of plants cause sickness in our bodies and people suffer from all forms of stomach distress and disease and all types of cancers. I am not saying that this is the only cause of cancer; there are many other factors which are important.

It seems most likely some of the main culprits which attribute to disease are Meat, Chicken, Pork and Fish. Let's take meat. Some may say meat is a very important food staple because it contains protein which is needed for the body to survive.

Yet there are some who disagree because with the advent of hormones, over the years the meat industry has been injecting growth hormones into their cattle which allow the cattle to put on more weight. This allows them to get a higher price for their meat.

These large meat companies are focused on growing cattle for this reason. In my estimation this is simple GREED. The investors and beef industry want to drown our any truthful words regarding growth hormones which are used in meat.

They are not concerned with the contamination of meats. Their only reason is to make a profit. Americans consume more chemicals in their food than any other nation in the world. It has been reported, every year 120 gallons of insecticides are being sprayed over our crops and no one is doing anything about it. The government sits, watching.

What is the solution? Do we go on eating meat? Is there another way to get our needed proteins? We can substitute beans, nuts, seeds and vegetables. Add oatmeal, broccoli, whole wheat and a great many more raw organic vegetables. The more fiber rich grains, fruits and vegetables we eat the more disease free we shall become. Where possible buy organic and look for only "no hormone/antibiotic" raised chicken, turkey, pork and fish.

Let's take Air for example. We need air to breathe and to survive. There are more and more automobiles on the roads today expelling carbon monoxide fumes; ever increasing daily. Carbon dioxide is a toxic gas which is odorless, tasteless and invisible. Airplanes, buses, trucks, and vans are also contributors. The burning of fossil fuel by organic manufacturers produces an extraordinary amount of toxic fumes into the atmosphere. This is why when we inhale toxic fumes the lungs along with the other

organs can become Cancerous.

Air pollution can be harmful to your health and can shorten life. Other pollutants are Radon gas in home basements, dust from wind, storms, and typhoons, decayed plants, house hold sprays, and cosmetic soaps. What is the solution? Eliminate toxic items mentioned from your everyday use. Rid yourself of the items you don't really need. Keep fumes down to a minimum, open all windows in the summer and welcome fresh air. The more you air out your rooms the cleaner the air will be.

The next factor which is necessary for one's survival is WATER. It is understood by many nutritionists and researchers that home tap water is loaded with unhealthy chemicals and gases: Chlorine, Fluorides, Copper, Lead, Chromium and Iron Salts. Our lakes, rivers and tributaries which run off into the oceans are loaded with toxic chemicals. Many of the chemicals are from manufacturers who produce chemicals found in laundry detergents, house cleaners, chlorine products, and all kinds of soaps.

Raw sewage from municipal processing plants, flowing into nearby rivers causes fish to die and changes the ecology of the ocean bed. Today 41% of the lake areas and 32% of the bays in the United States are polluted with high amounts of undesirable chemicals which can kill and stimulate the cells to proliferate into cancer cells. The cells making up our bodies required a pure clean system without these added toxic elements. One can see how important water is needed for survival. Buy bottled water which is considered a better choice than tap water.

Next is SOIL. Without clean pure unadulterated soil the food which we eat can kill us and cause all sorts of intestinal diseases including cancer. There are many books printed on the subject showing how the earth over the years has been contaminated with chemicals, insecticides and herbicides. The soil has been depleted of its necessary vitamins, minerals and nutrients, most importantly Selenium, a necessary mineral for plant life.

Worms need vitamins and minerals to reproduce. With unhealthy toxic soil, worms cannot exist or reproduce. If the soil is not turned over by worms the soil dries out and plants cannot live in a

dry clay hard soil. In some cases if plants do survive they absorb insecticides and herbicides. Consumers who purchase this food ingest the chemicals and suffer stomach and blood infections. It has been reported that millions of gallons of insecticides are sprayed over crops; oranges, corn and vegetables daily. This is definitely considered a serious factor in the spread of cancer.

How do we stop the ever continuing pollution by greedy investors who are more concerned with earnings rather than the safety of American lives?

The Solution: Contact our Representatives. Voice our opinions and concerns and make sure our AIR, WATER, and SOIL are free from pollutants.

28 FISH

The next food which is high in protein is fish. This protein contains omega 3 which has been highly linked to protecting against heart disease, breast cancers and other cancers, and relief of autoimmune diseases. High levels of omega 3 have been linked to extending the telomeres which extend one's life span. The longer the telomeres the longer the cells live.

There are two types of fish grown; the first is "farm raised" which in my estimation is feed food derived from local soil which is contaminated with insecticides and pesticides. Thus making fish food given to farm raised fish dangerous and toxic to humans.

The other which is considered best is wild fish, such as wild salmon and wild cod. Any wild fish is better than farm grown. Both fish mentioned above contain both omega 3, vitamins A,B, D and B12, amino acids and minerals. If you are planning to eat fish, choose wild salmon or wild cod.

Most large super grocery chains have a fish counter. Most of the fish being sold is frozen even though they say it's fresh. Avoid shell fish to an extent for they contain a great degree of mercury. The deeper the fish is in the ocean the greater the percentage of mercury it has. Watch very carefully how the fish appears. Has it turned color, from white to brown? Or does it have a very white color which might be from the lime water which is added on the fish to keep it looking fresh. There are many tricks to fool the public to buying fish that has turned somewhat uneatable but can be saved with a little trickery.

If in doubt about the fish leave it alone and go on your way for it is wiser to leave it. Don't buy fish just because it is inexpensive and looks fresh. The best telomere fish to eat is Alaskan Wild Salmon, Stripe Bass, Pacific Halibut, Wild Pollock and Pacific Cod.

29 FASTING EXTENDING LONGEVITY

Fasting is the cure all of all cure-alls. It is good to lower your blood pressure, it will prevent the enlargement of the prostate gland, help normalize the insulin and sugar content within the blood especially beneficial to type two diabetic sufferers. It will stimulate the phagocytes within the blood and help improve the immune stem. Relax your internal organs giving them a vacation for a while.

It will prevent diseases of the bowels and prevent irritable bowel syndrome. The list goes on and on. Fasting will help persons who suffer from asthma, emphysema, lung diseases, rectal irritations, hemorrhoids, and the like.

If you are considering fasting for more than a day, please contact your doctor and work along with his advice. For if you take it upon yourself to fast and if you're taking medication prescribed by your doctor it might conflict with the medicines you are taking and cause more harm than good. I don`t think one day a week would cause you any trouble. Yet, if you are considering fasting for more than a week, contact your doctor.

First thing in the morning, drink your fruit juice if you're not a diabetic. A good full glass. Then you can have a very small amount of low salt, low sugar yogurt and a cup of green tea. In the afternoon, a small amount of fruit along with ice tea. Nothing else.

In the evening time two glasses of water along with some mineral water. Nothing else. Fasting is the best medicine for not only your body but for your soul. Make fasting part of your health plan if you intend to lose weight.

30 SOME NEW TECHNOLOGIES

Would you believe me if I told you today we have new technologies which can grow new organs? Well believe me, scientists and researchers have discovered new technology in the production of heart and arteries and organs in general. Not from fetal stem cells, but from the persons own bone tissues. These cells are taken from a patient's bone marrow placed in a petri dish and multiplied. Then they are injected into a patient's heart to grow and repair the damage. This same procedure has been used in cases of PAD (patients who suffer from Peripheral arterial disease). These early studies have also suggested stem cells can reduce the number of amputations and help wounds heal by generating new blood supply to the affected limbs. These are in the third phase and are awaiting approval by the FDA.

Artificial Retina: This procedure is where a tiny video camera in the patients glasses captures a scene. Then the video is sent by way of the cable to a mini computer, where it is transformed into instructions which are sent back to the glasses. The instructions are then sent to an implant over the patients damaged retina. The implant emits signals which the brain interprets as images. This is also very new and awaits the FDA approval.

New Blood Thinner: Doctors and patients have been waiting for a new blood thinning drug which does not need monthly blood test monitoring. It in a limited way is a substitute for Warfarin a drug with many side effects and hard to control with blood tests. The new drug is called Pradaxa is considered 35 percent better than Warfarin. Yet it is only prescribed and approved for the treatment of patients who have had heart diseases not for patients who have PAD peripheral arterial diseases and pulmonary embolisms.

It is being used today with limited use. This drug must also be monitored every so often to determine the effect upon the patient's blood, including red and white blood cells.

Prostate Cancer Vaccine: Researchers are using a new vaccine known as Provenge. In this vaccine doctors remove some of the white blood cells from the patient and expose them to a protein found in prostate cancer and then they are injected back into the body where they prime the immune system to attack the cancer. This drug Provenge does not cure prostate cancer, but is found to reduce patient's overall risk of death by 24 percent.

There have been reported side effects, such as, chills, fever, headache, joint aches, and back pain but these usually disappear with a few days as reported by Dana Farber Institute in Boston, Mass. This drug was approved in 201 for cancer patients who have their cancer metastasized and have stopped responding to hormone treatments.

Growing one's own organs: It has been researched by a Doctor Anthony Atalo, in his laboratory has developed a shaped scaffolding strands of white muscle tissue contract in a lab dish. Then they have built biodegradable scaffolding shaped like a bladder, seeded with bladder and muscle cells from patients and implanted it into the person's body. It has had good results wherein the new bladder took over the functioning of the old cancerous bladder.

This work is promised to improve where other organs can be replaced with the same technique as practiced by Doctor Anthony Atalo at the Wake Forest Institute for regenerative medicine, in Winston, Salem North Carolina. Who would think within our lifetime we would see this to become possible? It will also extend our life span and who knows give us an edge on the cure of all diseases.

Robotics: This word is derived from a Czech writer Karec Capek in 1921. Robot comes from a Slavic word Robota which refers to forced labor. Robotics refers to a branch of science that deals with design, construction, and manufacturing of mechanical robots. How are robots applied today? They are applied as robotic artificial arms, legs, fingers, and toes. They can be uses both in commercial and domestic use. Domestically they can be used to drive tractors, work picking crops, digging and spreading top soil. Commercially, today there are planes made from mechanical parts driven by humans. Autos and trucks are also robots driven by humans. Tomorrow we will see robots driving trucks, planes and autos and will be amazed at what lies ahead for us.

What will robots be used for in the future? They will become care givers for the sick. They will be substitute nurses and will take vital signs of patients and report the results by the way of computers which are implanted within their systems. They will be used to quench fires and to walk into blazing fires to rescue victims.

Robots used in the military as tank drivers run by solders with computers and robots firing missiles, machine guns, flying radio control planes and a lot more army facilities. As cooks, messengers, workers, carpenters and replacing soldier's duties. Robots someday will speak and converse with humans. Use of facial expressions, artificial tears and emotions. A whole panorama of events shall be unfolded, amazing everyone. Not a science fiction ideology but a realistic science proven technology.

Conclusion: Scientists working with Robotics, Nanobiotics and Geometric Engineering will in the future be able to alleviate most of our diseases and will contribute to the extension of life well beyond our dreams.

Here are listed what is in sight for robots within the next ten to fifteen years.

- Robotic voice
- Facial expressions
- Artificial tears
- Artificial emotions
- Control in performing tasks

Another technology to consider is Nanotechnology (Nanotech). This is the manipulating matter on an atomic and molecular scale (Nano scale) which involves dimensions much smaller than a piece of human hair. Researchers have used Nanobits (particles) injected into guinea pigs and have followed the Nanobits as it travels throughout the blood stream. A monitor outside the body obtains an electrical signal from the Nanobit which can decipher diseased cells and organs. The early discovery of these cells can be treated before the cells metastasize preventing future intervention of radiation, chemotherapy or surgery.

It has been reported Nanotech could form molecular structures which might be used to regenerate human organs and body parts. With Nanotechnology and Robotics we may able to have robots act like humans and replace caregivers for the sick and handicapped. The amalgamation of Nanotech and robotics seems very possible in the near future. Nanobits can be used in computers, IPods and in electrical circuit boards replacing diodes and resistors. This technology is already being used in cosmetics, sunscreens and is opening up new phases of products such as batteries and electrical equipment.

The American Cancer Institute has created the Alliance for Nanotechnology in Cancer with the hope for investments in Nano Medicine leading to better drugs in the treatment of various forms of cancer.

To obtain additional information on Nanotech go to:

www.NanotechnologyandMedicin/Nanotechnologymedical applications.com

GENETIC ENGINEERING: Another important technology which is used in medicine and can be a cure for diseases and in extending life is the process of genetic engineering. What is genetic engineering? The process is the manipulation of those genes which are part of the DNA strains in such a way as to alter its numerical values either by substituting new numbers or changing existing numbers as to either cure or cause diseases. This method has been used to clone animals. We can also find from the DNA, which has four molecules, nucleotides (N), cytosine (C), adenine (A), guanine (G), thymine (T), each cross link with another and create a copy of itself into a single strain RNA molecule. The RNA communicates to the DNA link to twenty amino acids to form proteins which make life bearable. Genetic scientists are trying to create new protein artificial DNA in expanding the genetic alphabet.

With the replication of new proteins and the creation of new numbers, cell death in human diseases can be halted. This process of gene manipulation and cloning raises moral and religious questions and will be controversial for years to come. Yet leading scientists affirm that this is another key factor in the arsenal of Cancer treatments. In the not too distant future

I believe every person will be able to alter their genes to control the spread of their disease.   This will have an impact on human life and society. Medicine will be focused on gene replications and gene engineering.

31 A WALK THROUGH THE SUPERMARKET

Let's visit to your supermarket and select the best foods to eat. We walk to the vegetable department where we will have a choice of either the non-organic vegetable or the organic vegetables. I suggest picking the organic ones which are much healthier for you and your family. A new law which was passed a few years ago in 2003 stipulates that all supermarkets are required by law to identify the country of origin of fruits by placing a sticker on each fruit. If you can't find the origin of the country or the sticker ask the grocery clerk he will let you know.

You now walk to the fish department and look over what type of fish you desire. The right fish is any fish which has been caught from the deep oceans, e.g., sockeye salmon or cod fish. Most of the farm raised fish has been fed processed food which has been treated with toxic chemicals and is unhealthy. Choose wisely. Farm raised fish are known to contain Mercury, a poisonous metal. We don't want Mercury in our bodies.

Next, pass by the meat department and look for meats that do not contain hormones and antibiotics. These substances have been injected into the beef and all meats in order to increase the weight of the beef and also to prevent infections. You should stay away from consuming meats because you don't need hormones in your body that can cause all kinds of cancers. You don't need antibiotics because they also can cause cellular dysfunctions. This also goes for all canned meats and all canned products. Eat whole foods and plenty of fresh organic greens.

Continue walking past the middle aisles and don't stop. Here you will see all varieties of cans labeled, sausages, fruits, vegetables, beans and many other products. Why should you avoid canned

goods? Because these cans have preservatives added especially High Fructose Corn Syrup which is a substance that can harm your internal organs, causing a high buildup of cholesterol in your body. Some cans have more than fifteen chemicals listed and definitely without reservation are well noted as toxic by the scientific researchers and other nutritional doctors.

We now walk to the milk aisle and select the best milk for our money. The best is organic milk without hormones and without antibiotics. If you are selecting eggs, the best is organic eggs from chickens which have not been injected with hormones and antibiotics and which have been raised in non-penned cages.

As far as ice cream, purchase ice cream that doesn't have High Fructose Corn Syrup, Hydrogenated Cottonseed and Corn oil listed on the label. Look for a list of dyes. Don't buy ice cream with dyes even if they are vegetable dyes. These substances can cause hardening of the arteries and increase your cholesterol levels.

We should finish our shopping in the bread aisle where we should select only bread that doesn't contain high fructose corn syrup. This substance is used to keep the bread fresh and to prevent spoilage, giving the bread longer shelf life. The majority of bread products found are loaded with sugar and salt to enhance the flavor of the bread. Bread bakers and distributors are not interested in whether the product is healthy or not to the customers. They are only interested in the sale of the bread and in preventing it from spoiling.

Read all labels. Don't believe all you hear or told by store clerks for they are employees of the store. Choose the right food and shop wisely. Remember, if what you read on the labels is confusing, forget about it. Don't buy it. If there are more than five chemicals listed, don't buy it.

BE A WISE SHOPPER. CHOOSE YOUR FOOD WITH CAUTION.

THE SELECTION OF GOOD NUTRITION AND YOUR HEALTH LIES IN YOUR OWN HANDS.

LET YOUR FOOD BE YOUR MEDICINE!

CANCER PRODUCING ADDITITIVES

BANNED COLOR ADDITIVES:

- Butter Yellow – Green 1
- Green 2, Green 3, Yellow 3, 4
- Red 1, 2, 4, 32
- Sudan
- Violet 1
- Cinamyl anthuvanlate
- Cobalt salts
- Coumarin
- Cyclamate
- Dethyl procarbonate
- Ethylene glycol
- Monochloracidic acid
- Nordihyudroqualacetic acid
- Oil of calamus
- Polyoxyethylene sterate
- Myr 45
- Safrole
- Thiourea

Attach this list to your refrigerator. Refer to this list from time to time. (Compliments of CARE FOR THE LIVING)

32 EPILOGUE

I have listed all the therapies which I believe to be of importance to anyone who is planning to adopt an alternative method or protocol in the treatment of cancer. I have not added too much information on any one therapy because there are over one hundred pages on each subject. When you pick a therapy and you are considering it, do some research on the computer. If you don't have a computer go to your public library and search out the topic you desire. The information you are getting may someday save your or someone else's life.

I also have shown, in order to help avoid getting cancer, one should purchase only organic foods, take vitamins, minerals enzymes and electrolytes. Also, get rid of chemicals in the home, including hair sprays and cosmetics which contribute to the development of cancer. Become aware of toxic chemicals in all consumer products. If you have trouble reading large chemical names, it is better not to purchase them.

The main culprits preventing the cure for cancer are definitely the manufacturers of the carcinogenic chemicals and the big drug companies. These companies control the lobbyists in Washington D.C. with generous amounts of money. In doing so they are preventing us, the consumer, from knowing what toxic chemicals are in our foods, products, water and in our environment.

Here is an excerpt from Dr. Samuel Epstein, who is an environmental professor emeritus of the University Of Illinois School Of Public Health. He believes the cancer establishment has failed to do the work in informing the public on the chemicals in our daily food.

In his book "The Politics of Cancer Revisited" he states, "The cancer establishment has failed to allocate minimal priorities to research on cancer prevention. It has also failed to provide Congress and the executive with well documented scientific evidence on avoidable causes of cancer that would enable development of corrective legislative and regulatory action. Nor have U.S. citizens been advised of such information which

remains buried in confidential government and industry files or are relatively inaccessible in the scientific literatures, to enable them to protect themselves. Even more, both government and the public have been misled by repeated claims that we are winning the war against cancer. These claims are based on extravagant and unfounded announcements of dramatic advances in conventional treatment, coupled with highly prejudicial and unfounded attacks on alternative therapies".

We can surmise by Dr. Epstein's quote, he has expressed what I believe to be evident regarding cancer and how our government has chosen to look the other way when big conglomerates such as the billion dollar pharmaceutical companies and chemical companies are getting away with unscrupulous underhanded practices.

After considering all the material, well over thousands of sheets of research regarding the cure of Cancer, I have come to the conclusion that cancer cannot be eradicated by the discovery of a cure by one scientist or researcher or one big pharmaceutical company. It will take a unification of all scientists, worldwide,

together under the auspices of the United Nations to study and find how cancer can be prevented before it develops.

Every country together, submitting all their data and scientific research will make a big difference in eradicating cancer forever. In the near future, I strongly believe if the world scientists can come together with their facts, share and work together then we can extend life well beyond our imagination and DIE NO MORE.

TOMORROW WILL NEVER COME

YESTERDAY HAS GONE

TODAY IS HERE

LIVE ONE DAY AT A TIME

33 CANCER CHEMICALS IN OUR FOODS

SUPPORT PROCONSUMER REFORMS

Americans have a right to be informed of carcinogenic and reproductive toxins added to household products, cosmetics and foods. It is essential in view of the rising cases of cancer today. Many Americans are not aware of the many toxic chemicals added to the consumer's foods.

Did you know today on in three Americans are stricken with cancer and one in four will die. We are told that we are winning the war on Cancer but many researches such as occupational and environmental doctors say "We are not winning the war on Cancer". Why? Because our foods such as meats, dairy products and all other consumer products are loaded with toxic chemicals.

Cancer prevention is the best policy and we should contact our representatives and voice our opinion demanding chemical manufacturers remove and phase out the many toxic chemicals they place in all our consume food; everything we eat with the exception of organic foods.

We must insist, we want to know what toxic chemicals are in our foods and they should be listed in large letters so everyone young and old can read them without the use of a magnifying glass.   Also protect and expand the Delancy amendment of the Food, Drug and Cosmetic Act to ensure it not only retains its original powers but also expands them to include consumer products and the workplace.

If we all write to our representatives and make it known we want to know what's in our food, then we will succeed in reducing the cancer statistics. If not we are left with a very bleak future and many more Americans will die. Only a total phase out and ban on the manufacture, use and disposal of carcinogenic chemicals is likely to reverse the burgeoning toll of childhood cancers.

34 TO BE ESTABLISHED:
A NON-PROFIT ORGANIZATION

This non-profit organization "Care for The Living" will be established to help the poor underprivileged cancer and neurological diseased patients with financial assistance and also those incurable diseased patients who live alone who are in need of companions. The organization will provide educational and financial assistance to patients to enhance their quality of life.

The organization will also provide the public with a substantial body of well documented information on avoidable causes of cancer and related diseases. The organization shall seek donations from the public to coordinate raffles and arrange public meetings to continue asking for donations to foster the purpose of the organization.

The mission is to prevent and cure cancer and to improve lives of patients who are living with cancer. Also support and dedicated in brining integrative oncology into the mainstream of cancer treatments. Many philanthropists donate millions of dollars to colleges in order to build basketball courts, hospital wings and to their dogs and cats. Yet in America the sickly underprivileged poor who are facing incurable and un-treatable diseases are not cared for properly.

BECOME A MEMBER.

SEND YOUR NAME AND ADDRESS BELOW.

NO COST OR OBLIGATION.

You may also contact me at: ralfomilione1@att.net.or

   YOU CAN ORDER A COPY OF THIS BOOK"DIE NO MORE" AT-AMAZON.COM BY RALPH MILIONE.B.S.PH.

35 References: - WEB SITES

Life without Bread, How a Carbohydrate diet can save your life. Keats Publishing, Chicago Illinois. Authors Christian B. Allan, P.H.D. and Wolfgang Lutz, M.D.

Safe Shoppers Bible, Authors, David Steinman and Samuel S. Epstein, M.D., Publisher: Inc, New York, N.Y.

Fight Aging—practical information on general and scientific information on extending life. www.fightaging.com

The Fantastic Voyage; Authors Ray Kurezweil, and Terry Grossman, M.D. Publisher: Penguin Group, New York, N.Y. 2005

The Immortality Edge: Secrets of your telomeres for a longer and healthier life. Authors, Michael Fosse M.D. P.H.D. and Greata Blackburn, David Woynarowski, M.D.

The Politics of Cancer Revisited; Author, Samuel S. Epstein, M.D., Publisher: East Ridge Press, Fremont Center, N.Y. 1998, Henry Reginary Co., Chicago, Illinois,Henry Reginary Co., Chicago, Illinois

Pelton Press, Mind Food and Smart Pills by T and R. Publishing Company, Poway, California, 2003

Organic Flax Seed Oil, Spectrum Naturals by Yeh, Hylipidemia, Effects of Garlic Extract in Vivo and din Vitro, Pg 32

Food Makes the Difference by Patricia Kane, P.H.D., Simon and Shuster, Inc. 1230 Avenue of the Americas, New York, NY, 10020

How to Save Your Teeth, Everest Publications, House Publishers, New York, NY, 10020

Permanent Remissions, Pocket Books, Simon and Shuster Inc, 1230 Avenue of the Americas, New York, NY 10020

Therapy on Aging and Regeneration, Reamstone Publishing Co., 1997

Staying Well In A Toxic World, Lawson Lynn, Noble Press, 213 Institute Place, Suite 508, Chicago, Illinois, 60610

Jehro Kloss, Back to Eden, Books. Publishing Co., Loma Linda, California, 92354 (1999)

The New Fit on Fat, by Covert Bailey, Houghton Mifflin Company, 214 Park Avenue So., New York, NY 10003

Giannini Marilyn, Food Allergy Cookbook, PO Box 1250, Rocklin, California 95670

Heinermann, John, Science of Herbal Medicine by World Publishing Company, (1999)

Brainken, Harrit B. P.H.D., Getting Up When You're Feeling Down, G. Putnam and Sons, 200 Madison Avenue, New York, NY 10010

Leck, Sybil, Herbs- Medicine and Mysticism by Fredericks, Carlton and Goodman, Low Blood Sugar and You by Constellation International, 51 Madison Avenue, NY, 10003

The Merck Manual 2002, on herbs and medical treatment by Merck Publishing Co. New York, N.Y.

Choi, Steve S. Royal Jelly, The Fountain of Youth, Health World, Sept, 1991

Chapman, J.B., M.D. and Pery, Edward L. M.D. The Biochemic Handbook, Forman Inc. 1976

Oxygen Loading Diseases, A Survey of 100 Cases, Biochemical Medicine and Metabolic Biology, 1987

Thomas, John, Young Again-How to Reverse the Aging Process, Plexus Press 2010

Flax Oil As a True Aid Against Heart Infarction, Cancer and Other Diseases, Author Dr. Johanna Budwig, Publisher: Apple Publishing Co., LTD, Vancouver, British Columbia, 2004; The Oil Protein Diet by Dr. Johanna Budwig, Publisher, same as above.

Dietary Factors and the Survival Of Women with Breast Carcinoma, Authors Holmes, J.M. Stampfer, G. Colditz, B. Rosner Hankinson, S.W. Willet, J. Manson et al. , Plasma Sex Steroid Hormone Levels and Risk of Breast Cancer in Postmenopausal Women" Journal of Natural Cancer Institute 90(1998), 12920-1299

Consumer Product Safety Commission (CPSC), www.ccpsc.gov. Consumer health line: 800-638-2772

Environmental Protection Agency (EPA), www.epa.gov. (Protecting the Environment)

Matthew Gillian N.D. Electrolytes the Spark of Life by Natures Publication (2002)

Lee, Lila, Antitumor Properties of Natural Progesterone, Earth Publishing (1999)

Wallach, Joel Dr. and Booner, Wm Diseases of the Exotic Animals Medicine and Surgical Management by William Samuel Publishing Co., Philadelphie, PA

Weerbech, Melvyn, Natural Influence on Ailments by Lines Press, Cooper Richard, P.H.D., High Energy Living, St. Martins Press, New York, NY 20003

Locke, Dr. Andrew, The Family Guide to Homeopathy, (NY, Firesider)

Ornish, Deane, M.D., Dr. Dean Ornish's Program to Reversing Heart Disease, NY Times (1993)

William Lindsay, You Can Live, Life Publication, Pollard, Oregon, 1989

Coca, Arthur, The Secrets in Building Your Basic Health, Stuart Publications Inc, Secaucus, N.J. 1901